CHAIR YOGA EXERCISES

FOR MEN OVER 50

Structured Guide with Easy Daily

Workouts to Build Strength, Balance,

and Flexibility for older men

By

VANESSA H. GOURDINE

TABLE OF CONTENT

SECTION I

CHAPTER 1

- OVERVIEW OF CHAIR YOGA FOR MEN OVER 50

Understanding Chair Yoga

CHAPTER 2

BENEFIT OF CHAIR YOGA

CHAPTER 3

- GETTING STARTED
- Choosing the Right Chair

CHAPTER 4

- NUTRITION TIPS FOR MEN OVER 50 PRACTICING CHAIR YOGA

SECTION II

CHAPTER 5

- Chair yoga poses
- Warm-up- Exercises
- Seated postures
- Core Strengthening
- Lower Body Flexibility:

* **Balance and stability**

SECTION III

CHAPTER 6

Introduction to the 4-Week Chair Yoga Program for Men Over 50
Week 1
Establishing Foundations
Week 2
Deepening Practice
Week 3
Intensifying Focus
Week 4
Culminating Mastery
CHAPTER 6
JOURNAL AND TRACKER USER GUIDE
CHAPTER 7
TRACKER AND JOURNAL

INTRODUCTION

In the quiet corner of his living room, John found himself facing an unexpected adversary: a persistent stiffness that seemed to have declared war on his joints. As a man over 50, John had always prided himself on his vitality, but lately, his body was staging a rebellion of sorts.

It was during one particularly frustrating morning, as he struggled to tie his shoelaces with an uncooperative back, that he stumbled upon an unlikely savior – a simple, unassuming chair.

Enter the world of "Chair Yoga for Men Over 50," a transformative journey designed precisely for individuals like John, who have felt the subtle yet relentless effects of aging on their bodies.

This book isn't just about yoga; it's a lifeline for those seeking to reclaim their flexibility, strength, and overall well-being without the need for complicated postures or gym memberships.

In the pages that follow, you'll discover the incredible power that lies within the humble chair. Imagine turning your favorite recliner into a sanctuary of rejuvenation, a space where every stretch, twist, and breath brings you closer to a more agile and energized version of yourself.

As we delve into the art of chair yoga, you'll find a tailored approach that addresses the unique concerns faced by men over 50 – a roadmap to not only alleviate those nagging aches and pains but to embrace a lifestyle that defies the limitations imposed by age.

This isn't just a fitness guide; it's a companion on your journey to rediscovering the joy of movement and the freedom to live life on your terms.

So, if you've ever found yourself hesitating before reaching for that dropped pen, struggling with stairs that never used to be a challenge, or simply yearning for the vigor of your younger years, "Chair Yoga for Men

Over 50" is the solution you've been searching for. Let the chair become your ally in this rejuvenating odyssey – because it's never too late to reclaim your vitality and rewrite the story of your well-lived life.

SECTION I

CHAPTER 1

OVERVIEW OF CHAIR YOGA FOR MEN OVER 50

As men gracefully step into their 50s and beyond, the quest for maintaining health and vitality becomes paramount. Chair Yoga emerges as a uniquely tailored solution, offering a holistic approach to physical fitness, flexibility, and mental well-being. This comprehensive overview delves into the essence of Chair Yoga for Men Over 50, exploring its principles, benefits, and practical considerations.

Understanding Chair Yoga

Chair Yoga is a modified form of traditional yoga that adapts poses and exercises to be performed while seated or using a chair for support. Designed with the specific needs of men over 50 in mind, this practice acknowledges the physical changes associated with aging and provides a gentle yet effective way to stay active.

Adaptability and Inclusivity

The beauty of Chair Yoga lies in its adaptability. Whether you're a seasoned yogi or a complete beginner, the practice can be tailored to accommodate various fitness levels and physical abilities. It is an inclusive approach that fosters a sense of empowerment, making yoga accessible to a broader audience.

Seated Poses and Modified Movements

The core of Chair Yoga involves a series of seated poses and modified movements that aim to enhance flexibility, strength, and balance. From gentle stretches to controlled breathing exercises, each movement is thoughtfully curated to address the specific concerns of men over 50, such as joint stiffness and reduced range of motion.

Benefits for Physical Well-Being

Chair Yoga provides a myriad of physical benefits. It promotes flexibility by encouraging a full range of motion, enhances core strength, improves posture, and supports joint health. The gentle nature of the practice makes it an ideal choice for those managing conditions like arthritis or recovering from injuries.

Mind-Body Connection

Beyond the physical, Chair Yoga places a strong emphasis on the mind-body connection. Mindful breathing techniques and relaxation exercises contribute to stress reduction, mental clarity, and an overall sense of well-being. This comprehensive strategy recognizes the interdependence between physical and mental well-being.

Convenience and Accessibility

One of the key advantages of Chair Yoga is its convenience. The practice can be done virtually anywhere – at home, in the office, or even during travel – with nothing more than a sturdy chair. This accessibility eliminates barriers to consistent practice, making it a feasible and sustainable addition to daily routines.

Community and Social Interaction

Participating in Chair Yoga classes or group sessions provides an opportunity for men over 50 to connect with like-minded individuals. The social aspect of these gatherings fosters a sense of community, offering emotional support, encouragement, and a shared journey towards improved health.

Chair Yoga for Men Over 50 is not merely a set of exercises; it is a philosophy that empowers individuals to embrace aging with grace and vitality.

Through its adaptability, physical benefits, and emphasis on the mind-body connection, Chair Yoga stands as a comprehensive wellness tool. So, take a seat, embark on this rejuvenating journey, and discover the transformative power of

Chair Yoga for a healthier, more vibrant life.

CHAPTER 2

BENEFIT OF CHAIR YOGA

As men gracefully enter the golden phase of life, a vital aspect often overlooked is the maintenance of physical well-being. The natural aging process brings about changes in the body, impacting flexibility, strength, and overall mobility.

Enter Chair Yoga for Men Over 50 – a transformative practice that not only addresses these concerns but also provides a holistic approach to wellness. Let's delve into the comprehensive benefits of incorporating chair yoga exercises into the daily routine for men navigating the golden years.

Gentle Physical Exercise

Chair yoga offers a gentle yet effective way to engage in physical activity, catering to the unique needs of men over 50. The seated poses and modified movements provide a low-impact alternative, reducing strain on joints while promoting flexibility and balance. This makes it an ideal starting point for those who may be dealing with arthritis, stiffness, or other age-related challenges.

Enhanced Flexibility and Range of Motion

Regular chair yoga practice encourages the body to move through a full range of motion. The gentle stretching involved helps to maintain and improve flexibility, preventing the stiffness that often accompanies aging. Men over 50 can experience increased ease in daily activities, such as bending, reaching, and twisting, leading to a more active and fulfilling lifestyle.

Improved Posture and Core Strength

Chair yoga emphasizes the importance of proper posture and engages the core muscles. Strengthening the core not only supports the spine but also contributes to better balance and stability. As men age, maintaining good posture becomes crucial for preventing back pain and enhancing overall physical confidence.

Stress Reduction and Mental Well-Being

Beyond the physical benefits, chair yoga places a strong emphasis on mindful breathing and relaxation techniques. Men over 50 often juggle various responsibilities, leading to increased stress levels. Chair yoga provides a sanctuary to unwind, fostering mental clarity, reducing stress, and promoting a sense of calmness and overall well-being.

Cardiovascular Health

Chair yoga can be adapted to include cardiovascular exercises, promoting heart health. Incorporating rhythmic movements and controlled breathing into the practice helps enhance circulation, potentially lowering the risk of cardiovascular issues that become more prevalent with age.

Social Connection

Engaging in chair yoga classes or group sessions provides an opportunity for men over 50 to connect with like-minded individuals. Social interaction is a vital component of overall well-being, offering emotional support and encouragement, fostering a sense of community and camaraderie.

Accessible Anywhere, Anytime

One of the most significant advantages of chair yoga is its accessibility. Whether at home, in the office, or during travel, all that's needed is a chair. This convenience eliminates barriers to consistent practice, making it a feasible and sustainable addition to daily routines.

Chair yoga for men over 50 is not just a form of exercise; it's a holistic approach to aging gracefully. By embracing the comprehensive benefits of chair yoga, individuals can reclaim their vitality, enjoying improved physical and mental well-being. So, take a seat, embark on this transformative journey, and rediscover the joy of movement and wellness in the golden years.

CHAPTER 3

GETTING STARTED

Choosing the Right Chair

When embarking on the enriching journey of Chair Yoga, the first step is selecting the right chair to support your practice. Not just any chair will suffice – you need one that provides stability, comfort, and adaptability. Here's a breakdown of considerations:

Stability and Durability

Opt for a chair with a solid and stable frame. The last thing you want during your yoga practice is an unstable foundation. Ensure that the chair can withstand your weight and movements without wobbling or tipping.

Seat Height

The ideal chair height allows your feet to rest comfortably on the floor, maintaining a stable base. If your chair is too high or too low, it can disrupt your alignment and compromise the effectiveness of the exercises. Consider chairs with adjustable height options for personalized comfort.

Armrests

While armrests are a common feature, they should not hinder your movements. Look for a chair with armrests that allow your arms to move freely during stretches and exercises. Some practitioners prefer chairs without armrests for unrestricted movement.

Back Support

A supportive backrest is crucial for maintaining good posture. Look for a chair with a straight back that supports the natural curvature of your spine. Chairs with adjustable lumbar support can be particularly beneficial.

Comfortable Seat Cushion

Your chair should have a comfortable seat cushion to make prolonged sitting more pleasant. However, the cushion should not be too soft, as it may hinder stability during certain poses.

Comfortable Clothing and Environment

Creating a conducive environment for your Chair Yoga practice goes beyond just the chair. Comfortable clothing and an inviting space can significantly enhance your experience.

Clothing Choice

Opt for loose, breathable clothing that allows for unrestricted movement. Stretchable fabrics are ideal, ensuring that you can comfortably transition between poses without any hindrance. Dress in layers, so you can adjust as needed to maintain a comfortable body temperature.

Creating a Yoga Space

Designate a quiet and clutter-free space for your Chair Yoga practice. This space doesn't need to be large – a corner of a room will suffice. Ensure there is ample natural light and good ventilation. Adding a few calming elements, such as plants or soothing colors, can contribute to a serene atmosphere.

Proper Ventilation

Yoga is a practice that involves controlled breathing, so a well-ventilated space is crucial. Ensure that your chosen practice area allows for fresh air circulation. If possible, practice near an open window or in a room with good airflow.

Adequate Lighting

Well-lit surroundings are essential for safety and focus during your practice. Natural light is ideal, but if that's not possible, ensure that your practice space is well-lit with artificial lighting that doesn't create harsh shadows.

By investing time in choosing the right chair and creating a comfortable practice environment, you lay the foundation for a fulfilling and effective Chair Yoga experience. As you step onto this path of well-being, remember that the journey begins with thoughtful choices and a commitment to your own health and vitality.

Setting the Right Mood

Creating an ambiance that aligns with the essence of yoga can significantly enhance your practice. Consider the following elements to set the right mood for your Chair Yoga sessions:

Music and Sounds

Select calming background music or nature sounds that resonate with you. Gentle instrumental tunes or soft nature sounds can create a soothing atmosphere, helping you relax and focus on your breath and movements.

Aromatherapy

Incorporate aromatherapy into your practice space by using essential oils or candles with calming scents. Lavender, chamomile, and eucalyptus are commonly chosen for their calming characteristics. A subtle aroma can elevate your practice and contribute to a tranquil environment.

Mindful Lighting

Consider using candles or soft, adjustable lighting to create a serene atmosphere. Dim lighting can help ease eye strain and induce a sense of calmness, allowing you to connect more deeply with your practice.

Preparing Your Mind

Before you start your Chair Yoga session, take a few moments to prepare your mind. The mental aspect of yoga is just as important as the physical.

Mindful Breathing

Sit comfortably in your chosen chair and focus on your breath. Take a deep breath through your nostrils, letting your belly expand, and release the breath gradually through your mouth. This mindful breathing not only calms the mind but also prepares you for the movements ahead.

Clearing Mental Clutter

Take a moment to release any mental clutter or stress. Acknowledge any thoughts that may be distracting you, and then gently let them go. Chair Yoga is a time for self-care, and this mental preparation ensures you can fully immerse yourself in the practice.

As you choose the right chair, create a comfortable environment, and set the mood for your practice, you're laying the groundwork for a fulfilling Chair Yoga journey. This holistic approach encompasses not only the physical but also the mental and emotional aspects of well-being. By investing in these initial steps, you are opening the door to a rejuvenating practice that will contribute to your health, vitality, and overall sense of balance. Get ready to experience the transformative power of Chair Yoga for men over 50.

CHAPTER 4

NUTRITION TIPS FOR MEN OVER 50 PRACTICING CHAIR YOGA

As men enter their 50s and beyond, maintaining a balanced and nutrient-rich diet becomes crucial for overall well-being. Combining the benefits of Chair Yoga with mindful nutrition creates a holistic approach to health. Let's explore essential nutrition tips, healthy eating habits, and nutrient-rich snack ideas tailored for men over 50 engaging in Chair Yoga.

Nutrition Tips for Chair Yoga Enthusiasts

Adequate Protein Intake

As the body ages, maintaining muscle mass becomes increasingly important. Ensure your diet includes sufficient protein, which is vital for muscle repair and maintenance. Opt for lean protein sources such as poultry, fish, beans, and dairy.

Hydration is Key

Proper hydration is essential for joint health and overall bodily functions. Aim for at least eight glasses of water a day, and consider incorporating hydrating foods like watermelon, cucumber, and herbal teas into your routine.

Balanced Nutrient Intake

Embrace a diverse and colorful array of fruits and vegetables to ensure you're getting a spectrum of essential nutrients. Include leafy greens, berries, citrus fruits, and cruciferous vegetables to support immune function, digestion, and heart health.

Mindful Portion Control

As metabolism tends to slow with age, practicing portion control is crucial. Focus on consuming balanced meals with a mix of carbohydrates, proteins, and healthy fats to sustain energy levels throughout the day.

Healthy Eating Habits for Men Over 50

Emphasize Whole Foods

Prioritize whole, minimally processed foods over highly refined options. Whole grains, lean proteins, and a variety of fruits and vegetables provide essential nutrients and fiber, contributing to digestive health.

Reduce Sodium Intake

Limiting sodium helps manage blood pressure and reduces the risk of cardiovascular issues. Opt for herbs and spices to flavor your meals instead of relying heavily on salt. Be cautious of processed foods, as they frequently possess elevated sodium levels.

Include healthy fat

Include sources of beneficial fats in your diet, such as avocados, nuts, seeds, and olive oil. These fats support brain health, joint function, and contribute to overall cardiovascular well-being.

Regular Meal Timing

Establishing regular meal times helps regulate metabolism and provides a steady source of energy. Aim for three balanced meals and, if needed, incorporate healthy snacks to curb hunger between meals.

Nutrient-Rich Snack Ideas

Greek Yogurt with Berries

Combine the protein-rich goodness of Greek yogurt with antioxidant-packed berries for a delicious and satisfying snack that supports muscle health and provides essential vitamins.

Nut and Seed Mix

Create a customized mix of almonds, walnuts, chia seeds, and pumpkin seeds for a nutrient-dense snack rich in omega-3 fatty acids and protein.

Sliced Apple with Nut Butter

Pair crisp apple slices with almond or peanut butter for a delightful combination of fiber, healthy fats, and a touch of sweetness.

Vegetable Sticks with Hummus

Enjoy the crunch of fresh carrot and cucumber sticks dipped in hummus for a satisfying, nutrient-packed snack that promotes digestive health.

Integrating these nutrition tips, healthy eating habits, and nutrient-rich snack ideas into your lifestyle complements the benefits of Chair Yoga for men over 50. Nourishing your body with wholesome foods not only supports your yoga practice but also contributes to sustained energy, enhanced flexibility, and overall vitality. As you embark on this holistic journey, savor the opportunity to nourish both your body and spirit, paving the way for a healthier and more fulfilling life.

SECTION II

CHAPTER 5

Chair yoga poses

Warm-up- Exercises

1. Seated Neck Rolls:

- Instructions:
    - Sit comfortably in the chair with your feet flat on the floor.
    - Inhale and lengthen your spine.
    - Breathe out and softly lower your chin towards your chest.

- o Inhale and roll your head to the right, bringing your right ear towards your right shoulder.
- o Exhale and continue the circular motion, rolling your head back and to the left.
- o Complete the circle, returning to the starting position.
- o Repeat in the opposite direction.
- o Do this for 1-2 minutes, breathing deeply and slowly.

2. Shoulder Rolls:

- Instructions:

- Sit with an upright posture and keep your shoulders at ease.

- Inhale while raising your shoulders towards your ears.

- Exhale and rotate your shoulders in a circular motion, moving them back and down.

- Repeat this sequence for 1-2 minutes, then switch to a forward roll.

- Concentrate on relieving tension in your shoulders and neck.

3. Wrist Circles:

- Instructions:

- o Extend your arms straight out in front of you.
- o Make fists with your hands and rotate your wrists in circular motions.
- o After 1-2 minutes, reverse the direction of the circles.
- o This helps improve flexibility and reduce stiffness in the wrists.

4. **Seated Side Stretch:**

- Instructions:
  - o Sit with your feet flat on the floor.
  - o Inhale and raise your arms overhead.

- Hold your left wrist with your right hand and gently lean to the right.
- Feel the stretch along your left side.
- Wait for 15 to 30 seconds before changing to the opposite side.
- Repeat 2-3 times on each side.

5. Seated Forward Bend:

- Instructions:
  - Sit with your feet flat on the floor and spine straight.
  - Inhale and lengthen your spine.

- o Exhale and hinge at your hips, reaching towards your toes.
- o Hold for 15-30 seconds, feeling the stretch in your lower back and hamstrings.
- o Inhale as you come back to an upright position.
- o Repeat 2-3 times.

6. Ankle Rolls:

- Instructions:
  - o Lift one foot off the floor and rotate your ankle in a circular motion.
  - o After 1-2 minutes, reverse the direction of the circles.

- Switch to the other ankle and repeat.
- This helps improve ankle flexibility and mobility.

7. Seated Cat-Cow Stretch:

- Instructions:
  - Take a seated position on the chair, ensuring your feet are firmly planted on the ground.
  - Inhale as you arch your back and raise your chest, mimicking the Cow pose.
  - Exhale while rounding your spine and bringing your chin towards your chest, imitating the Cat pose.

- Continue this fluid sequence for 1-2 minutes, synchronizing the movements with your breath.

8. Seated Hip Opener:

- Instructions:
    - Take a comfortable seated position with both feet resting flat on the floor. Specifically, cross your left ankle over your right knee to create a figure-four shape.
    - Inhale deeply while elongating your spine, feeling a gentle stretch in your left hip. Hold this pose for 15-30

seconds, then switch to the other side.

  - Repeat this sequence 2-3 times on both sides for a well-rounded stretch.

9. Seated Twist:

- Instructions:

  - Sit comfortably with your feet grounded on the floor and ensure your spine remains straight.

  - Inhale deeply, extending your back. Exhale as you gently twist to the right, placing your left hand on your right knee and your right hand on the back of the chair for support.

- o Hold the twist for 15-30 seconds, breathing deeply. Repeat this twisting sequence on the opposite side.
- o Aim to complete 2-3 sets on each side for a comprehensive stretch.

10. **Deep Breathing Exercise:**

- Instructions:
    - o Find a comfortable seated position with both feet resting flat on the floor.
    - o Close your eyes and inhale deeply through your nostrils.

- Exhale gradually through your mouth, concentrating on completely releasing the air from your lungs.
- Engage in deep breathing for a duration of 2-3 minutes, letting your body unwind and relax.

Seated postures

1. Chair Mountain Pose:

Instructions:

- Sit comfortably with feet firmly grounded.
- Inhale deeply, lifting your arms above with

palms facing each other.

- Stretch your spine and hold for 15-30 seconds.
- Exhale, bringing arms down; repeat 2-3 times.

2. Seated Forward Bend:

Instructions:

- Sit with feet flat, spine straight.

- Inhale, raise arms, exhale, tilt forward.
- Use chair edges for support.
- Hold for 15-30 seconds, repeating 2-3 times

3. Twist with Side Stretch:

Instructions;

- Sit with flat feet, inhale, raise arms.

- Exhale, twist right, left hand on right knee.
- Inhale, stretch spine; exhale, reach right arm left.
- Hold for 15-30s, switch sides; repeat 2-3 times.

4. Cat-Cow Stretch:

Instructions:

- Sit at the chair edge, feet flat.

- Inhale, arch back (Cow); exhale, tuck chin (Cat).
- Flow for 1-2 minutes in sync with breath.

5. Seated Pigeon Pose:

Instructions

- Sit, lift right leg, place ankle on left knee.
- Inhale, stretch spine; exhale, lean forward.

- Hold 15-30s, switch sides; repeat 2-3 times.

6. Eagle Arms:

Instructions :

- Sit, feet flat, inhale, stretch arms.
- Exhale, cross right arm over left, palms together.
- Hold 15-30s, feel stretch; repeat on left.

- Do 2-3 sets on each side.

7. Butterfly Stretch:

- Sit, feet together, knees bent out.
- Inhale, stretch spine; exhale, press knees down.
- Hold 15-30s, feel inner thigh stretch; repeat 2-3 times.

8. Seated Warrior Pose:

Sit, feet flat, lift right knee.

Hold right knee, extend left arm back.

Hold 15-30s, switch sides; repeat 2-3 times..

9. Side Leg Lifts:

- Sit straight, feet flat.
- Inhale, lift right leg to side.
- Hold, engage outer hip; exhale, lower.
- Repeat on the left; aim for 10-15 reps.

10. Seated Boat Pose:

- Sit on the chair edge, feet flat.
- Inhale, elevate legs, forming a V.
- Hold for 15-30s; exhale, lower.
- Repeat 2-3 times.

Core Strengthening:

1. Seated Knee Lifts:

Instructions

- Position yourself at the edge of the chair with your feet flat.
- Grasp the sides of the chair, elevate your right knee, and exhale as you lower it; repeat with the left.
- Aim to complete 10-15 lifts for each leg.

2. Russian Twists:

Instructions

- Sit with your feet flat and spine straight,

holding onto the chair sides.

- Inhale, stretch your spine, and exhale while twisting your torso to the right.

- Return to the center with an inhale, then repeat the twist on the left.

- Complete 2-3 sets on each side.

3. Extensions with Crunch:

Instructions

- Maintain a seated position with feet flat and spine straight, holding the chair sides.
- Inhale, extend your right leg, and exhale while bringing the knee to your chest, performing a crunch.
- Inhale to extend the leg and repeat as necessary.

4. Seated Bicycle Crunches:

Instructions

- Sit with your feet flat, spine straight, and hold onto the chair for support.

- Lift your feet slightly, inhale, and bring the right knee toward your chest while twisting to the left.

- Exhale, switch sides, bringing the left knee towards the chest while turning to the right.

- Continue in a bicycle motion for 1-2 minutes.

5. Seated Side Plank:

Instructions

- Sit on the chair's edge
  with feet together,
  placing your right hand
  on the chair.

- Inhale, elevate your
  hips, and stretch your
  left arm towards the
  ceiling.

- Hold for 15-30
  seconds, engaging your

core, then exhale and lower your hips.

- Perform the same action on the opposite side, repeating for 2-3 sets.

6. Seated Boat Pose:

Instructions

- Sit near the chair's edge, feet flat, and hold onto the sides for support.
- Inhale, elevate your legs, forming a V shape

with your torso, and engage your core.

- Hold for 15-30 seconds, exhale, and lower your legs; repeat 2-3

times.

7. Seated Leg Lifts:

Instructions

- Sit on the chair's edge with feet flat, holding onto the sides.
- Inhale, lift both legs straight out, engage

your lower abdominals, and hold for a moment.

- Exhale, lower your legs, and repeat for 10-15 repetitions.

8. Seated Reverse Crunches:

- Sit with feet flat, spine straight, and hold onto the chair sides.

- Inhale, lift your knees towards your chest, rounding your spine.

- Exhale, lower your feet back towards the floor; repeat for 10-15 reps.

9. Seated Windshield Wipers:

Instructions

- Sit with feet flat, holding the chair sides for support.
- Inhale, lift your knees to your chest, exhale, and lower them to the right.
- Inhale back to center, exhale, and lower to the left; repeat for 1-2 minutes.

10. Seated Core Twist with Leg Extension:

Instructions

- Sit with feet flat and spine straight, holding the chair sides.

- Inhale, lift your right knee towards your chest, exhale, twist your torso to the right, and stretch your right leg out.

- Inhale back to the center, repeat on the left; aim for 10-15 reps on each side.

Lower Body Flexibility

1. Chair Seated Forward Bend:

Instructions

- Sit on the chair with feet flat, inhale to stretch your spine.
- Exhale, hinge at the hips, reaching towards your toes.
- Hold 15-30 seconds, feeling hamstrings and lower back.
- Inhale, return upright; repeat 2-3 times.

2. Seated Butterfly Stretch:

Instructions

- Sit with straight back, soles together.
- Hold feet; inhale, stretch spine.
- Exhale, press knees towards floor.
- Hold 15-30 seconds, feeling inner thighs.
- Repeat 2-3 times..

3. Seated Leg Cross Stretch:

Instructions

- Sit, legs extended.
- Cross right ankle over left.
- Inhale, stretch spine.
- Exhale, bend forward, reaching towards toes.
- Hold 15-30 seconds, feel stretch in outer hip and thigh.

- Inhale, sit back up; switch legs; repeat 2-3 times on each side..

4. Seated Knee to Chest Stretch:

Instructions

- Sit, feet flat.
- Lift right knee towards chest.
- Hug knee; hold 15-30 seconds, stretch in hip and lower back.

- Release, switch to left knee.
- Repeat 2-3 times on each side.

5 Seated Hamstring Stretch:

Instructions

- Sit, right leg extended, left foot against inner thigh.
- Inhale, stretch spine.
- Exhale, hinge at hips, reaching towards right toes.

- Hold 15-30 seconds, feeling stretch in right hamstring.
  - Inhale, sit back up; switch legs; repeat 2-3 times on each side..

6. **Seated Hip Opener:**

Instructions

- Sit, feet flat.

- Cross right ankle over left knee (figure-four shape).
- Inhale, stretch spine.
- Exhale, lean forward, stretch in right hip.
- Hold 15-30 seconds, switch sides; repeat 2-3 times..

7. Seated Figure-Four Stretch:

- Sit, feet flat.
- Cross right ankle over left knee.
- Inhale, sit tall.

- Exhale, press down on right knee, stretch in outer hip.
- Hold 15-30 seconds, switch sides; repeat 2-3 times.

8. Seated Calf Stretch:

Instructions

- Sit, feet flat.
- Extend right leg, flex foot.
- Inhale, flex foot.
- Exhale, press on ball of foot, stretch in calf.

- Hold 15-30 seconds, switch sides; repeat 2-3 times.

9. Seated Ankle Rolls:

Instructions

- Sit, feet flat.
- Lift one foot, rotate ankle in circles.
- After 1-2 minutes, reverse circles.
- Switch to other ankle; repeat.

10. Seated Straddle Stretch:

- Sit with legs wide.

- Inhale, stretch spine.

- Exhale, tilt forward at hips.

- Hold 15-30 seconds, feeling inner thighs and hamstrings.

- Inhale, return upright; repeat 2-3 times.

Remember to move deliberately, breathing deeply throughout each stretch. If discomfort arises, ease out and consult a healthcare expert.

Balance and stability

1. **Seated Mountain Pose:**
   - Sit comfortably, feet flat.
   - Ground feet, stretch spine.
   - Palms together at chest.
   - Hold 15-30s, focusing on breath.
   - Release, repeat 2-3 times.
2. **Seated Leg Lifts with Arm Extension:**
   - Sit, feet flat.
   - Inhale, lift right leg, stretch left arm.
   - Hold, engage core.
   - Exhale, lower leg and arm.
   - Repeat on other side.
   - Aim for 10-15 reps each side.
3. **Seated Tree Pose:**
   - Sit, feet flat.

- Lift right foot, place on inner left thigh.
- Palms together at chest.
- Hold 15-30s, focus on balance.
- Release, repeat on the other side.
- Repeat 2-3 times each side.

4. Seated Side Leg Lifts:

- Sit with straight back, feet flat.
- Inhale, lift right leg to side.
- Hold, engage the outer hip.
- Exhale, lower leg.
- Repeat on left.
- Aim for 10-15 reps each leg.

5. Seated Figure-Four Stretch with Twist:

- o Sit, feet flat.
- o Cross right ankle over left knee.
- o Inhale, sit tall.
- o Exhale, twist to the right.
- o Hold 15-30s, engage core.
- o Release, repeat on other side.
- o Repeat 2-3 times each side.

6. Seated Warrior III:

- o Sit at chair edge, feet flat.
- o Extend right leg straight back.
- o Reach arms forward, parallel to floor.
- o Hold 15-30s, engage core.
- o Lower right foot, repeat on left.
- o Aim for 2-3 sets each side.

7. **Seated Heel Raises:**

   - Sit comfortably, feet flat.

   - Inhale, lift both heels.

   - Hold, engage calf muscles.

   - Exhale, lower heels.

   - Repeat for 10-15 reps.

8. **Seated Warrior II:**

   - Sit, feet flat, legs wide.

   - Turn right foot right, stretch arms parallel to floor.

   - Engage core, hold 15-30s.

   - Release, repeat on left.

   - Aim for 2-3 sets each side.

9. **Seated Side Plank:**

   - Sit, feet together.

   - Right hand on chair, lift hips.

   - Stretch left arm towards ceiling.

- o Hold 15-30s, engage core.
- o Exhale, lower hips.
- o Repeat on other side.
- o Do 2-3 sets each side.

10. **Seated Balancing Twist:**

- o Sit comfortably, feet flat.
- o Inhale, stretch spine.
- o Exhale, twist right, left hand on right knee.
- o Hold 15-30s, engage core.
- o Inhale to center, repeat on left.
- o Do 2-3 sets each side.

Remember to move with control, focus on breath, and use the chair for support when needed. Adjust positions if discomfort arises, and consult a healthcare expert if necessary.

SECTION III

CHAPTER 6

Introduction to the 4-Week Chair Yoga Program for Men Over 50

Embrace a journey of strength, flexibility, and holistic well-being with our Chair Yoga Exercises tailored for men over 50. In this section, we present a comprehensive 4-week workout plan crafted to seamlessly integrate into your daily routine. Curated exercises from distinct categories - Warm-Up, Seated Postures, Core Strengthening, Lower Body Flexibility, and Balance & Stability - form the foundation of this transformative program.

Week 1 & 2: Establishing Foundations with Warm-Up Exercises (Category: Warm-Up Exercises)

- *Morning:* Energize your mornings with seated neck rolls and shoulder rolls, invigorating your body for the day ahead.
- *Evening:* Wind down gracefully with seated cat-cow stretches and wrist circles, promoting flexibility and relaxation.

Week 3 & 4: Deepening Practice with Seated Postures (Category: Seated Postures)

- *Morning:* Foster lower body flexibility with seated leg lifts and ankle rolls, enhancing mobility and strength.
- *Evening:* Cultivate balance and stability with seated tree poses and seated side leg lifts, promoting overall well-being.

Core Strengthening Emphasis (Category: Core Strengthening)

- *Morning:* Start your day with seated knee lifts and seated Russian twists, activating and strengthening your core.

- *Evening:* Conclude your day with seated leg extensions with crunches and seated bicycle crunches, enhancing core strength and stability.

Lower Body Flexibility Focus (Category: Lower Body Flexibility)

- *Morning:* Improve hamstring flexibility with seated hamstring stretches, ensuring a strong and flexible lower body.

- *Evening:* Enhance hip mobility with seated pigeon poses and seated figure-four stretches, promoting overall lower body flexibility.

Balance and Stability Integration (Category: Balance and Stability)

- *Morning:* Strengthen your core and improve stability with seated boat poses and seated warrior II poses.
- *Evening:* Promote balance with seated side plank poses and seated balancing twists, enhancing overall stability.

In addition to this meticulously designed workout plan, you'll find a recording journal and tracker. The journal invites you to reflect on your journey, while the tracker serves as a guide, ensuring you stay aligned with your fitness goals.

As we navigate through these four weeks together, Chair Yoga becomes a powerful tool to rejuvenate both the body and mind. Let's embark on this transformative path, unlocking the full potential of chair yoga for a healthier, more resilient you.

Week 1

Establishing Foundations

Day 1:

- *Morning:*
  1. Warm-Up Exercise (A): Seated Neck Rolls
     - *Criteria:* Gentle neck mobility and relaxation.
     - *Duration:* 1 minute (30 seconds each direction).
  2. Balance and Stability (E): Seated Tree Poses
     - *Criteria:* Enhancing balance and stability.

- ■ *Duration:* Hold each side for 30 seconds.
- *Evening:*
  1. Core Strengthening (C): Seated Knee Lifts
     - ■ *Criteria:* Activating and strengthening the core.
     - ■ *Count:* 15 lifts on each leg.
  2. Lower Body Flexibility (D): Seated Hamstring Stretches
     - ■ *Criteria:* Improving hamstring flexibility.
     - ■ *Duration:* Hold for 30 seconds on each leg.

Day 2:

- *Morning:*

    1. Warm-Up Exercise (A): Seated Shoulder Rolls

        - *Criteria:* Loosening shoulder tension and promoting flexibility.

        - *Count:* 15 rolls forward and 15 rolls backward.

    2. Seated Posture (B): Seated Leg Lifts

        - *Criteria:* Promoting lower body flexibility and strength.

        - *Count:* 10 lifts on each leg.

- *Evening:*

    1. Core Strengthening (C): Seated Russian Twists

- *Criteria:* Engaging and strengthening the core.
- *Count:* 20 twists (10 on each side).

2. Balance and Stability (E): Seated Side Leg Lifts

- *Criteria:* Enhancing stability and strengthening the outer hips.
- *Count:* 12 lifts on each leg.

Day 3:

- *Morning:*

1. Warm-Up Exercise (A): Seated Wrist Circles

- *Criteria:* Easing wrist tension and promoting joint flexibility.
- *Count:* 20 circles in each direction.

2. Seated Posture (B): Seated Forward Bend

- *Criteria:* Enhancing flexibility in the lower back and hamstrings.
- *Duration:* Hold for 30 seconds, reaching towards your toes.

- *Evening:*

1. Core Strengthening (C): Seated Leg Extensions with Crunch

- ■ *Criteria:* Activating the core and promoting strength.
- ■ *Count:* 12 extensions with crunches.

2. Lower Body Flexibility (D): Seated Pigeon Poses

- ■ *Criteria:* Stretching and opening the hips.
- ■ *Duration:* Wait for 30 seconds on each side.

Day 4:

- ● *Morning:*

1. Warm-Up Exercise (A): Seated Ankle Rolls

- **Criteria:** Improving ankle flexibility and mobility.
- **Count:** 15 rolls in each direction.

2. Balance and Stability (E): Seated Warrior II Poses
    - **Criteria:** Promoting balance and strength in the lower body.
    - **Duration:** Hold each side for 30 seconds.

- *Evening:*
    1. Core Strengthening (C): Seated Bicycle Crunches
        - **Criteria:** Engaging the core muscles and promoting flexibility.

- *Count:* 20 bicycle crunches (10 on each side).

2. Balance and Stability (E): Seated Balancing Twists

   - *Criteria:* Enhancing balance and stability.

   - *Duration:* Hold each side for 30 seconds.

Day 5:

- *Morning:*

   1. Warm-Up Exercise (A): Seated Side Neck Stretches

      - *Criteria:* Easing tension in the neck and shoulders.

- *Duration:* Hold each side for 20 seconds.

2. Seated Posture (B): Seated Butterfly Stretch

   - *Criteria:* Promoting flexibility in the inner thighs.

   - *Duration:* Hold for 30 seconds, gently pressing knees towards the floor.

- *Evening:*

  1. Core Strengthening (C): Seated Reverse Crunches

     - *Criteria:* Targeting the lower abdominal muscles.

- **Count:** 15 reverse crunches.

2. Lower Body Flexibility (D): Seated Leg Lifts

   - *Criteria:* Enhancing flexibility in the legs and hips.
   - *Count:* 10 lifts on each leg.

Day 6:

- *Morning:*

  1. Warm-Up Exercise (A): Seated Side Twists

     - *Criteria:* Warming up the spine and improving flexibility.

- *Count:* 15 twists on each side.

2. Balance and Stability (E): Seated Boat Poses

   - *Criteria:* Engaging the core and promoting stability.

   - *Duration:* Hold for 20 seconds, lifting the legs to a comfortable height.

- *Evening:*

  1. Core Strengthening (C): Seated Windshield Wipers

     - *Criteria:* Activating the core and improving flexibility.

     - *Count:* 12 rotations (6 on each side).

2. Balance and Stability (E):
Seated Side Plank

- *Criteria:* Promoting core strength and overall stability.

- *Duration:* Hold for 20 seconds on each side.

Day 7:

- *Morning:*

1. Warm-Up Exercise (A):
Seated Full Body Stretch

- *Criteria:* Waking up the entire body and increasing overall flexibility.

- *Duration:* Hold for 30 seconds, reaching arms

overhead and pointing toes.

2. Seated Posture (B): Seated Knee to Chest Stretch

   - *Criteria:* Stretching the lower back and promoting flexibility.
   - *Duration:* Hold each knee for 20 seconds.

- *Evening:*

  1. Core Strengthening (C): Seated Boat Poses

     - *Criteria:* Engaging the core and promoting overall stability.
     - *Duration:* Hold for 25 seconds.

2. Lower Body Flexibility (D):
Seated Figure-Four Stretch

- *Criteria:* Stretching the outer hips and promoting flexibility.
- *Duration:* Hold each side for 25 seconds.

Week 2

Deepening Practice

Day 8:

- *Morning:*
    1. Warm-Up Exercise (A): Seated Arm Circles

- *Criteria:* Increasing circulation and warming up the arms.
    - *Count:* 20 circles forward and 20 circles backward.
2. Balance and Stability (E): Seated Side Plank
    - *Criteria:* Enhancing core strength and promoting stability.
    - *Duration:* Hold for 25 seconds on each side.

- *Evening:*
    1. Core Strengthening (C): Seated Leg Lifts with Arm Extension

- **Criteria:** Engaging the core and improving overall strength.
        - **Count:** 12 lifts on each leg.
    2. Balance and Stability (E): Seated Warrior II Poses
        - **Criteria:** Promoting balance and strength in the lower body.
        - **Duration:** Hold each side for 25 seconds.

Day 9:

- *Morning:*
    1. Warm-Up Exercise (A): Seated Shoulder Blade Squeezes

- *Criteria:* Relieving tension in the shoulders and upper back.
- *Count:* 15 squeezes, focusing on contracting and relaxing the shoulder blades.

2. Seated Posture (B): Seated Cross-Legged Stretch
    - *Criteria:* Opening up the hips and stretching the inner thighs.
    - *Duration:* Hold for 30 seconds, gently pressing knees towards the floor.

- *Evening:*

1. Core Strengthening (C):
   Seated Boat Poses

   - *Criteria:* Engaging the
     core and promoting
     overall stability.

   - *Duration:* Hold for 25
     seconds.

2. Lower Body Flexibility (D):
   Seated Figure-Four Stretch

   - *Criteria:* Stretching the
     outer hips and
     promoting flexibility.

   - *Duration:* Hold each
     side for 25 seconds.

Day 10:

- *Morning:*

1. Warm-Up Exercise (A): Seated Full Body Stretch

    - *Criteria:* Waking up the entire body and increasing overall flexibility.

    - *Duration:* Hold for 30 seconds, reaching arms overhead and pointing toes.

2. Seated Posture (B): Seated Knee to Chest Stretch

    - *Criteria:* Stretching the lower back and promoting flexibility.

    - *Duration:* Hold each knee for 25 seconds.

- *Evening:*

1. Core Strengthening (C): Seated Russian Twists

   - *Criteria:* Engaging and strengthening the core.
   - *Count:* 25 twists (12 on each side).

2. Balance and Stability (E): Seated Side Plank

   - *Criteria:* Promoting core strength and overall stability.
   - *Duration:* Hold for 25 seconds on each side.

Day 11:

- *Morning:*

   1. Warm-Up Exercise (A): Seated Side Neck Stretches

- *Criteria:* Easing tension in the neck and shoulders.
    - *Duration:* Hold each side for 25 seconds.

2. Seated Posture (B): Seated Butterfly Stretch
    - *Criteria:* Promoting flexibility in the inner thighs.
    - *Duration:* Hold for 30 seconds, gently pressing knees towards the floor.

- *Evening:*

1. Core Strengthening (C): Seated Reverse Crunches

- *Criteria:* Targeting the lower abdominal muscles.
- *Count:* 18 reverse crunches.

2. Lower Body Flexibility (D): Seated Leg Lifts

- *Criteria:* Enhancing flexibility in the legs and hips.
- *Count:* 12 lifts on each leg.

Day 12:

- *Morning:*

    1. Warm-Up Exercise (A): Seated Side Twists

- *Criteria:* Warming up the spine and improving flexibility.
    - *Count:* 18 twists on each side.
2. Balance and Stability (E): Seated Boat Poses
    - *Criteria:* Engaging the core and promoting stability.
    - *Duration:* Hold for 22 seconds, lifting the legs to a comfortable height.
- *Evening:*
    1. Core Strengthening (C): Seated Windshield Wipers

- *Criteria:* Activating the core and improving flexibility.
- *Count:* 15 rotations (8 on each side).

2. Balance and Stability (E): Seated Side Plank

- *Criteria:* Promoting core strength and overall stability.
- *Duration:* Hold for 22 seconds on each side.

Day 13:

- *Morning:*

   1. Warm-Up Exercise (A): Seated Full Body Stretch

- *Criteria:* Waking up the entire body and increasing overall flexibility.
    - *Duration:* Hold for 30 seconds, reaching arms overhead and pointing toes.

2. Seated Posture (B): Seated Knee to Chest Stretch
    - *Criteria:* Stretching the lower back and promoting flexibility.
    - *Duration:* Hold each knee for 25 seconds.

- *Evening:*

    1. Core Strengthening (C): Seated Bicycle Crunches

- **Criteria:** Engaging the core muscles and promoting flexibility.
- **Count:** 20 bicycle crunches (10 on each side).

2. Balance and Stability (E): Seated Balancing Twists

- **Criteria:** Enhancing balance and stability.
- **Duration:** Hold each side for 25 seconds.

Day 14:

- *Morning:*

1. Warm-Up Exercise (A): Seated AnkleCircles

- *Criteria:* Improving ankle flexibility and mobility.
- *Count:* 20 circles in each direction.

■ Seated Posture (B): Seated Forward Bend with Side Reach

- *Criteria:* Enhancing flexibility in the lower back and sides.
- *Duration:* Hold for 30 seconds, alternating side reaches.

2. *Evening:*

- Core Strengthening (C): Seated Leg Cross Crunches
  - *Criteria:* Engaging the core and targeting oblique muscles.
  - *Count:* 15 cross crunches on each side.
- Lower Body Flexibility (D): Seated Wide-Legged Stretch
  - *Criteria:* Stretching the inner thighs and

promoting
flexibility.

- *Duration:* Hold
  for 30 seconds,
  reaching towards
  the floor.

Week 3

Intensifying Focus

Day 15:

- *Morning:*

    1. Warm-Up Exercise (A): Seated Side Neck Stretches

        - *Criteria:* Easing tension in the neck and shoulders.

        - *Duration:* Hold each side for 25 seconds.

    2. Seated Posture (B): Seated Butterfly Stretch

- *Criteria:* Promoting flexibility in the inner thighs.
- *Duration:* Hold for 30 seconds, gently pressing knees towards the floor.

- *Evening:*
  1. Core Strengthening (C): Seated Reverse Crunches
     - *Criteria:* Targeting the lower abdominal muscles.
     - *Count:* 18 reverse crunches.
  2. Lower Body Flexibility (D): Seated Leg Lifts

- *Criteria:* Enhancing flexibility in the legs and hips.
- *Count:* 12 lifts on each leg.

Day 16:

- *Morning:*

  1. Warm-Up Exercise (A): Seated Side Twists
     - *Criteria:* Warming up the spine and improving flexibility.
     - *Count:* 18 twists on each side.
  2. Balance and Stability (E): Seated Boat Poses

- *Criteria:* Engaging the core and promoting stability.
  - *Duration:* Hold for 22 seconds, lifting the legs to a comfortable height.
- *Evening:*
  1. Core Strengthening (C): Seated Windshield Wipers
     - *Criteria:* Activating the core and improving flexibility.
     - *Count:* 15 rotations (8 on each side).
  2. Balance and Stability (E): Seated Side Plank

- **Criteria:** Promoting core strength and overall stability.
- **Duration:** Hold for 22 seconds on each side.

Day 17:

- *Morning:*

  1. Warm-Up Exercise (A): Seated Full Body Stretch
     - **Criteria:** Waking up the entire body and increasing overall flexibility.
     - **Duration:** Hold for 30 seconds, reaching arms overhead and pointing toes.

2. Seated Posture (B): Seated Knee to Chest Stretch

- *Criteria:* Stretching the lower back and promoting flexibility.
- *Duration:* Hold each knee for 25 seconds.

- *Evening:*

1. Core Strengthening (C): Seated Bicycle Crunches

- *Criteria:* Engaging the core muscles and promoting flexibility.
- *Count:* 20 bicycle crunches (10 on each side).

2. Balance and Stability (E): Seated Balancing Twists

- ■ *Criteria:* Enhancing balance and stability.
- ■ *Duration:* Hold each side for 25 seconds.

Day 18:

- ● *Morning:*
    1. Warm-Up Exercise (A): Seated Ankle Circles
        - ■ *Criteria:* Improving ankle flexibility and mobility.
        - ■ *Count:* 20 circles in each direction.
    2. Seated Posture (B): Seated Forward Bend with Side Reach

- ■ *Criteria:* Enhancing flexibility in the lower back and sides.
  - ■ *Duration:* Hold for 30 seconds, alternating side reaches.

- *Evening:*
  1. Core Strengthening (C): Seated Leg Cross Crunches
     - ■ *Criteria:* Engaging the core and targeting oblique muscles.
     - ■ *Count:* 15 cross crunches on each side.
  2. Lower Body Flexibility (D): Seated Wide-Legged Stretch

  - *Criteria:* Stretching the inner thighs and promoting flexibility.
  - *Duration:* Hold for 30 seconds, reaching towards the floor.

Day 19:

- *Morning:*

  1. Warm-Up Exercise (A): Seated Neck Rolls
     - *Criteria:* Gentle neck mobility and relaxation.
     - *Duration:* 1 minute (30 seconds each direction).

  2. Balance and Stability (E): Seated Tree Poses

- *Criteria:* Enhancing balance and stability.
- *Duration:* Hold each side for 30 seconds.

- *Evening:*
  1. Core Strengthening (C): Seated Knee Lifts
     - *Criteria:* Activating and strengthening the core.
     - *Count:* 15 lifts on each leg.
  2. Lower Body Flexibility (D): Seated Hamstring Stretches
     - *Criteria:* Improving hamstring flexibility.
     - *Duration:* Hold for 30 seconds on each leg.

Day 20:

- *Morning:*

  1. Warm-Up Exercise (A): Seated Shoulder Rolls
     - *Criteria:* Loosening shoulder tension and promoting flexibility.
     - *Count:* 15 rolls forward and 15 rolls backward.
  2. Seated Posture (B): Seated Leg Lifts
     - *Criteria:* Promoting lower body flexibility and strength.
     - *Count:* 10 lifts on each leg.

- *Evening:*

1. Core Strengthening (C): Seated Russian Twists

   - *Criteria:* Engaging and strengthening the core.
   - *Count:* 20 twists (10 on each side).

2. Balance and Stability (E): Seated Side Leg Lifts

   - *Criteria:* Enhancing stability and strengthening the outer hips.
   - *Count:* 12 lifts on each leg.

Day 21:

- *Morning:*

1. Warm-Up Exercise (A): Seated Wrist Circles

   - *Criteria:* Easing wrist tension and promoting joint flexibility.
   - *Count:* 20 circles in each direction.

2. Seated Posture (B): Seated Forward Bend

   - *Criteria:* Enhancing flexibility in the lower back and hamstrings.
   - *Duration:* Hold for 30 seconds, reaching towards your toes.

- *Evening:*

1. Core Strengthening (C): Seated Leg Extensions with Crunch

   - *Criteria:* Activating the core and promoting strength.
   - *Count:* 12 extensions with crunches.

2. Lower Body Flexibility (D): Seated Pigeon Poses

   - *Criteria:* Stretching and opening the hips.
   - *Duration:* Wait for 30 seconds on both sides.

This completes Day 21 of Week 3. If you'd like to continue with the remaining days of Week 3 and proceed to Week 4, please let me know.

Week 4

Culminating Mastery

Day 22:

- *Morning:*

    1. Warm-Up Exercise (A): Seated Side Neck Stretches

        - *Criteria:* Easing tension in the neck and shoulders.

        - *Duration:* Hold each side for 25 seconds.

2. Seated Posture (B): Seated
   Butterfly Stretch

   - *Criteria:* Promoting
     flexibility in the inner
     thighs.

   - *Duration:* Hold for 30
     seconds, gently
     pressing knees towards
     the floor.

- *Evening:*

  1. Core Strengthening (C):
     Seated Reverse Crunches

     - *Criteria:* Targeting the
       lower abdominal
       muscles.

     - *Count:* 18 reverse
       crunches.

2. Lower Body Flexibility (D): Seated Leg Lifts

- *Criteria:* Enhancing flexibility in the legs and hips.
- *Count:* 12 lifts on each leg.

Day 23:

- *Morning:*

  1. Warm-Up Exercise (A): Seated Side Twists

     - *Criteria:* Warming up the spine and improving flexibility.
     - *Count:* 18 twists on each side.

2. Balance and Stability (E): Seated Boat Poses

- *Criteria:* Engaging the core and promoting stability.
- *Duration:* Hold for 22 seconds, lifting the legs to a comfortable height.

- *Evening:*

  1. Core Strengthening (C): Seated Windshield Wipers

     - *Criteria:* Activating the core and improving flexibility.
     - *Count:* 15 rotations (8 on each side).

  2. Balance and Stability (E): Seated Side Plank

- *Criteria:* Promoting core strength and overall stability.
- *Duration:* Hold for 22 seconds on each side.

Day 24:

- *Morning:*

  1. Warm-Up Exercise (A): Seated Full Body Stretch
     - *Criteria:* Waking up the entire body and increasing overall flexibility.
     - *Duration:* Hold for 30 seconds, reaching arms overhead and pointing toes.

2. Seated Posture (B): Seated Knee to Chest Stretch

- ■ *Criteria:* Stretching the lower back and promoting flexibility.
- ■ *Duration:* Hold each knee for 25 seconds.

- *Evening:*

1. Core Strengthening (C): Seated Bicycle Crunches

- ■ *Criteria:* Engaging the core muscles and promoting flexibility.
- ■ *Count:* 20 bicycle crunches (10 on each side).

2. Balance and Stability (E): Seated Balancing Twists

- **Criteria:** Enhancing balance and stability.
- **Duration:** Hold each side for 25 seconds.

Day 25:

- *Morning:*

    1. Warm-Up Exercise (A): Seated Ankle Circles
        - **Criteria:** Improving ankle flexibility and mobility.
        - **Count:** 20 circles in each direction.
    2. Seated Posture (B): Seated Forward Bend with Side Reach

- *Criteria:* Enhancing flexibility in the lower back and sides.
- *Duration:* Hold for 30 seconds, alternating side reaches.

- *Evening:*
  1. Core Strengthening (C): Seated Leg Cross Crunches
     - *Criteria:* Engaging the core and targeting oblique muscles.
     - *Count:* 15 cross crunches on each side.
  2. Lower Body Flexibility (D): Seated Wide-Legged Stretch

- *Criteria:* Stretching the inner thighs and promoting flexibility.
- *Duration:* Hold for 30 seconds, reaching towards the floor.

Day 26:

- *Morning:*

    1. Warm-Up Exercise (A): Seated Neck Rolls

        - *Criteria:* Gentle neck mobility and relaxation.
        - *Duration:* 1 minute (30 seconds each direction).

    2. Balance and Stability (E): Seated Tree Poses

- *Criteria:* Enhancing balance and stability.
  - *Duration:* Hold each side for 30 seconds.

- *Evening:*
  1. Core Strengthening (C): Seated Knee Lifts
     - *Criteria:* Activating and strengthening the core.
     - *Count:* 15 lifts on each leg.
  2. Lower Body Flexibility (D): Seated Hamstring Stretches
     - *Criteria:* Improving hamstring flexibility.
     - *Duration:* Hold for 30 seconds on each leg.

Day 27:

- *Morning:*

    1. Warm-Up Exercise (A): Seated Shoulder Rolls
        - *Criteria:* Loosening shoulder tension and promoting flexibility.
        - *Count:* 15 rolls forward and 15 rolls backward.
    2. Seated Posture (B): Seated Leg Lifts
        - *Criteria:* Promoting lower body flexibility and strength.
        - *Count:* 10 lifts on each leg.

- *Evening:*

1. Core Strengthening (C): Seated Russian Twists

   - ■ *Criteria:* Engaging and strengthening the core.
   - ■ *Count:* 20 twists (10 on each side).

2. Balance and Stability (E): Seated Side Leg Lifts

   - ■ *Criteria:* Enhancing stability and strengthening the outer hips.
   - ■ *Count:* 12 lifts on each leg.

Day 28:

- *Morning:*

1. Warm-Up Exercise (A): Seated Wrist Circles

    - *Criteria:* Easing wrist tension and promoting joint flexibility.
    - *Count:* 20 circles in each direction.

2. Seated Posture (B): Seated Forward Bend

    - *Criteria:* Enhancing flexibility in the lower back and hamstrings.
    - *Duration:* Hold for 30 seconds, reaching towards your toes.

- *Evening:*

1. **Core Strengthening (C):**
   Seated Leg Extensions with
   Crunch

   - *Criteria:* Activating the
     core and promoting
     strength.

   - *Count:* 12 extensions
     with crunches.

2. **Lower Body Flexibility (D):**
   Seated Pigeon Poses

   - *Criteria:* Stretching
     and opening the hips.

   - *Duration:* Wait for 30
     seconds on both sides.

Day 29:

- *Morning:*

1. Warm-Up Exercise (A):
    Seated Side Neck Stretches

    - *Criteria:* Easing
      tension in the neck and
      shoulders.
    - *Duration:* Hold each
      side for 25 seconds.

2. Seated Posture (B): Seated
    Butterfly Stretch

    - *Criteria:* Promoting
      flexibility in the inner
      thighs.
    - *Duration:* Hold for 30
      seconds, gently
      pressing knees towards
      the floor.

- *Evening:*

1. Core Strengthening (C): Seated Bicycle Crunches

   - *Criteria:* Engaging the core muscles and promoting flexibility.
   - *Count:* 20 bicycle crunches (10 on each side).

2. Balance and Stability (E): Seated Balancing Twists

   - *Criteria:* Enhancing balance and stability.
   - *Duration:* Hold each side for 25 seconds.

Day 30: Final Day Celebration!

- *Morning and Evening:*
  - Choose Your Favorites:

- *Select your favorite warm-up, seated posture, core strengthening, lower body flexibility, and balance and stability exercises from the past month.*

- *Complete each exercise with a sense of accomplishment and mindfulness.*

- *Duration and count as per your comfort.*

Congratulations on completing the 30-day Chair Yoga for Men Over 50 program! If you have enjoyed the journey and wish to continue, feel free to revisit any of your preferred exercises or explore new variations. Remember, consistency is key to reaping the full benefits of your practice. Wishing you continued wellness and vitality!

CHAPTER 6

JOURNAL AND TRACKER USER GUIDE

Welcome to the Chair Yoga Exercises for Men over 50 Journal and Tracker User Guide! This guide is designed to support your chair yoga journey over the next 4 weeks. Inside, you'll find exercise trackers to record your workouts and reflection pages to document your thoughts and progress.

The exercise tracker is a valuable tool, providing designated spaces for each day, morning and evening sessions, and checkboxes to mark off completed exercises. This structured layout will help you stay organized and visualize your daily accomplishments, fostering a sense of achievement.

Following each week's tracker, you'll discover reflection pages. These pages serve as a canvas for documenting challenges, milestones, motivation, and the emotions tied to your chair yoga practice. Engaging in this reflective dialogue allows you to connect with your past, present, and future selves, serving as a testament to your unwavering dedication.

To extend your chair yoga practice beyond the initial 4 weeks, we've included additional tracker and reflection pages. This journal is more than just a book; it symbolizes your commitment to fitness and the boundless possibilities that lie ahead. Let it serve as a motivational tool, encouraging you to maintain consistency and celebrate your achievements throughout your chair yoga journey.

Embrace the transformative power of chair yoga and use this Journal and Tracker User Guide as your companion in achieving wellness and vitality. May it inspire you to thrive on the path of chair yoga exercises tailored for men over 50.

CHAPTER 7

TRACKER AND JOURNAL

DAYS	EXERCISES	CHECK

REFLECTION

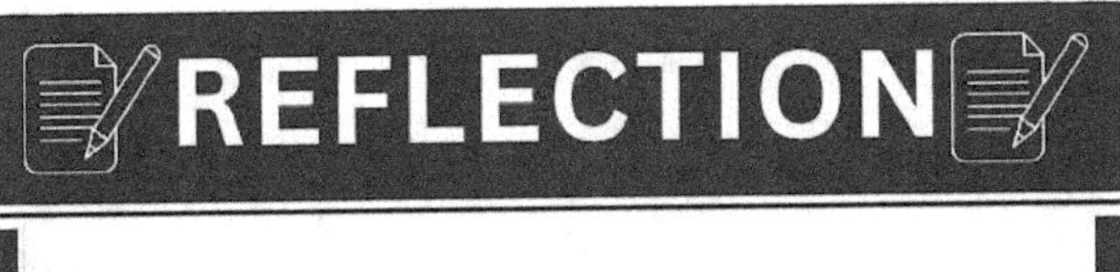

REFLECTION

REFLECTION

DAYS	EXERCISES	CHECK

REFLECTION

REFLECTION

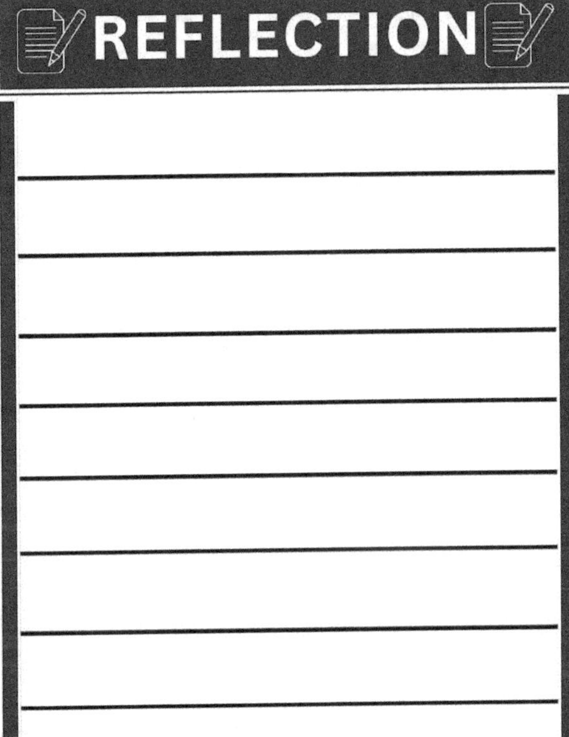

REFLECTION

DAYS	EXERCISES	CHECK

REFLECTION

REFLECTION

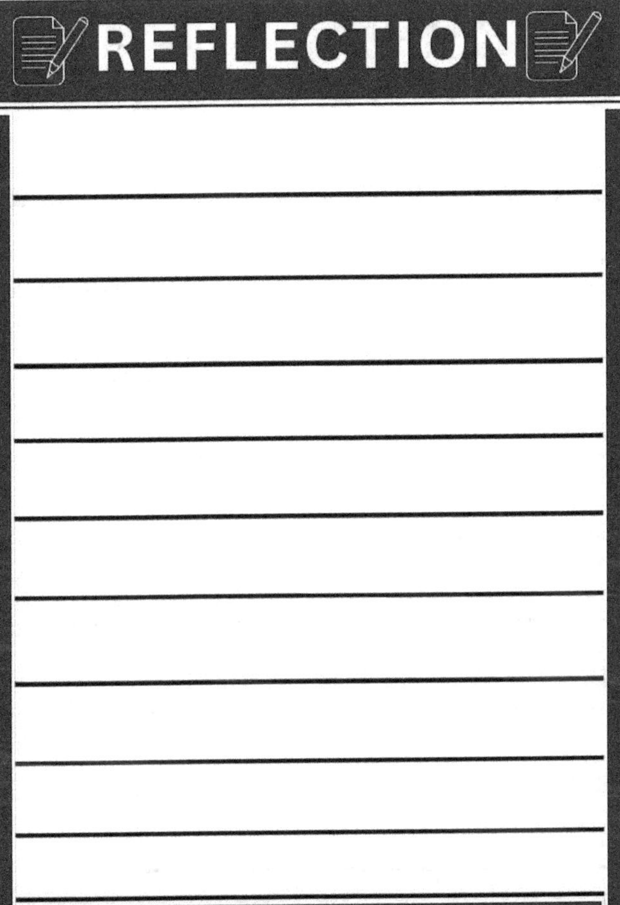

REFLECTION

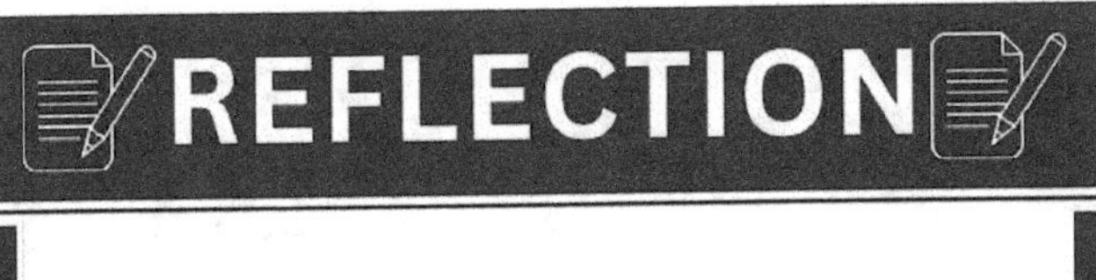

DAYS	EXERCISES	CHECK

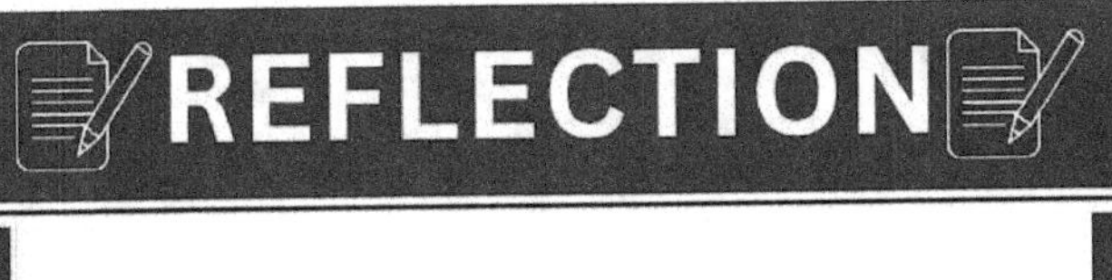

REFLECTION

REFLECTION

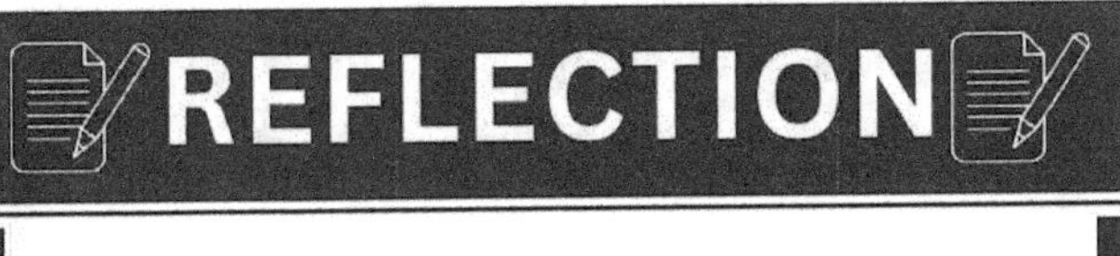

REFLECTION

REFLECTION